Title: Croctober: Time Savings - Volume Five

by Jenny Koo

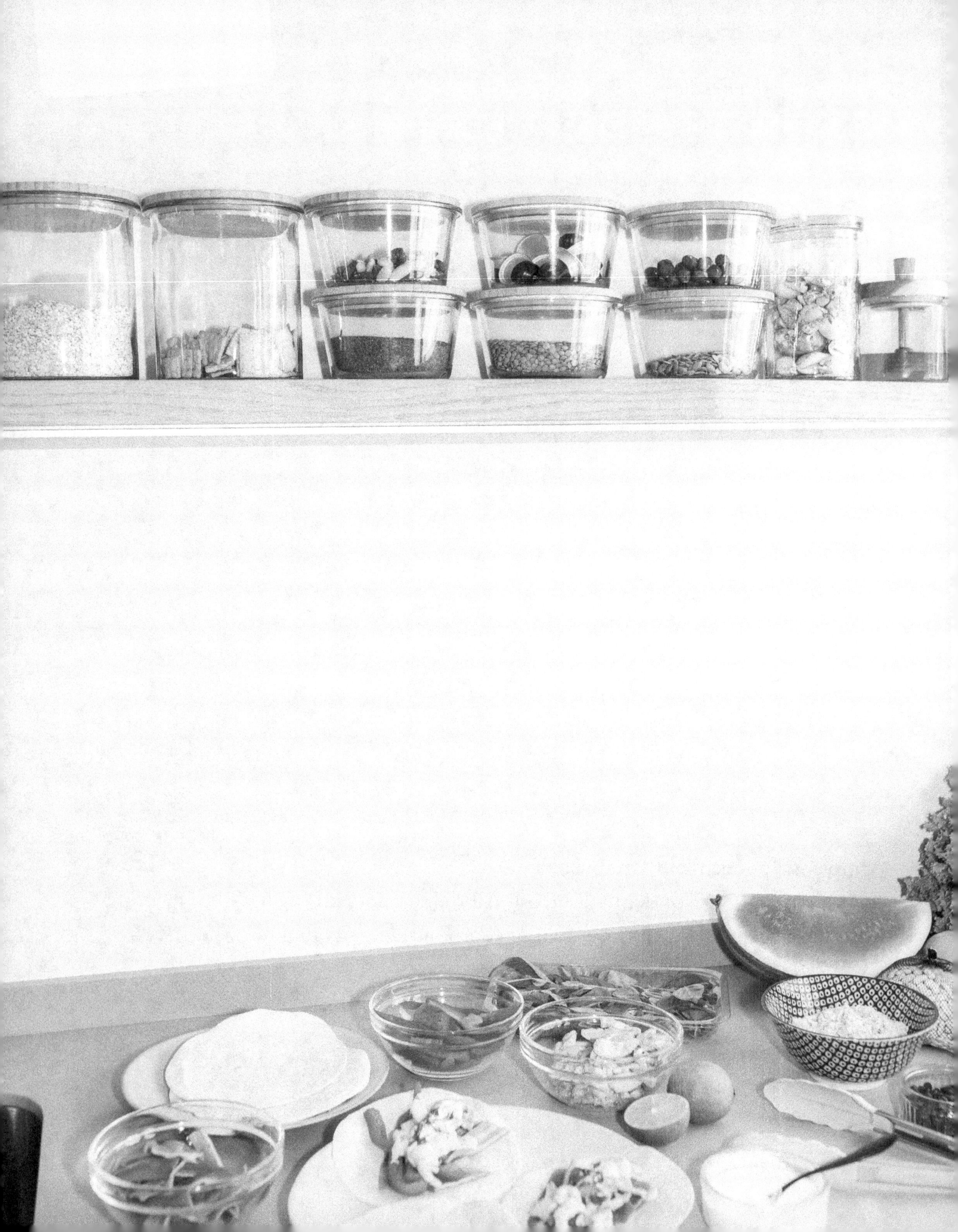

Title: Croctober: Time Savings - Volume Five

Introduction:

- Briefly introduce the concept of the "Time Savings" series.
- Emphasize the focus on quick and efficient crockpot cooking.
- Encourage readers to explore the time-saving recipes in this volume.

Chapter 1: Quick and Easy Breakfasts

- Overnight Oats with Berries
- Crockpot Breakfast Casserole
- Apple Cinnamon Porridge
- Veggie Omelette
- Blueberry French Toast

Chapter 2: Effortless Soups and Stews

- Hearty Chicken Noodle Soup
- Vegetable Lentil Soup
- Beef and Barley Stew
- Sweet Potato and Black Bean Chili
- Creamy Tomato Basil Soup

Chapter 3: Speedy Chicken Dishes

- Lemon Garlic Chicken
- Honey Sriracha Chicken
- BBQ Pulled Chicken
- Chicken and Rice Casserole
- Creamy Chicken Alfredo

Chapter 4: Time-Efficient Beef and Pork Creations

- Beef and Broccoli Stir Fry
- Classic Pot Roast
- BBQ Pork Ribs
- Beef and Vegetable Soup
- Teriyaki Beef Tips

Chapter 5: Rapid Seafood Meals

- Lemon Butter Garlic Shrimp
- Crockpot Salmon with Herbs
- Spicy Seafood Gumbo
- Clam Chowder
- Tilapia with Mediterranean Veggies

These recipes are designed to save time while creating delicious meals using a crockpot. Each recipe serves 4 to 5 people and includes a list of ingredients, nutrition benefits, approximate calories per serving, and step-by-step instructions for ease of preparation.

Conclusion:

- Summarize the variety of time-saving crockpot recipes included in this volume.
- Encourage readers to enjoy quick and delicious meals not only during Croctober but throughout the year.

Bonus Section: Create Your Own Recipes!

We Include Blank Recipe Cards Templates and Notes Sections for Your Own Cooking Journals. Be Creative. Explore the Endless Possibilities and Create Your Own. Feel Free to Reproduce the Templates for your Own Use.

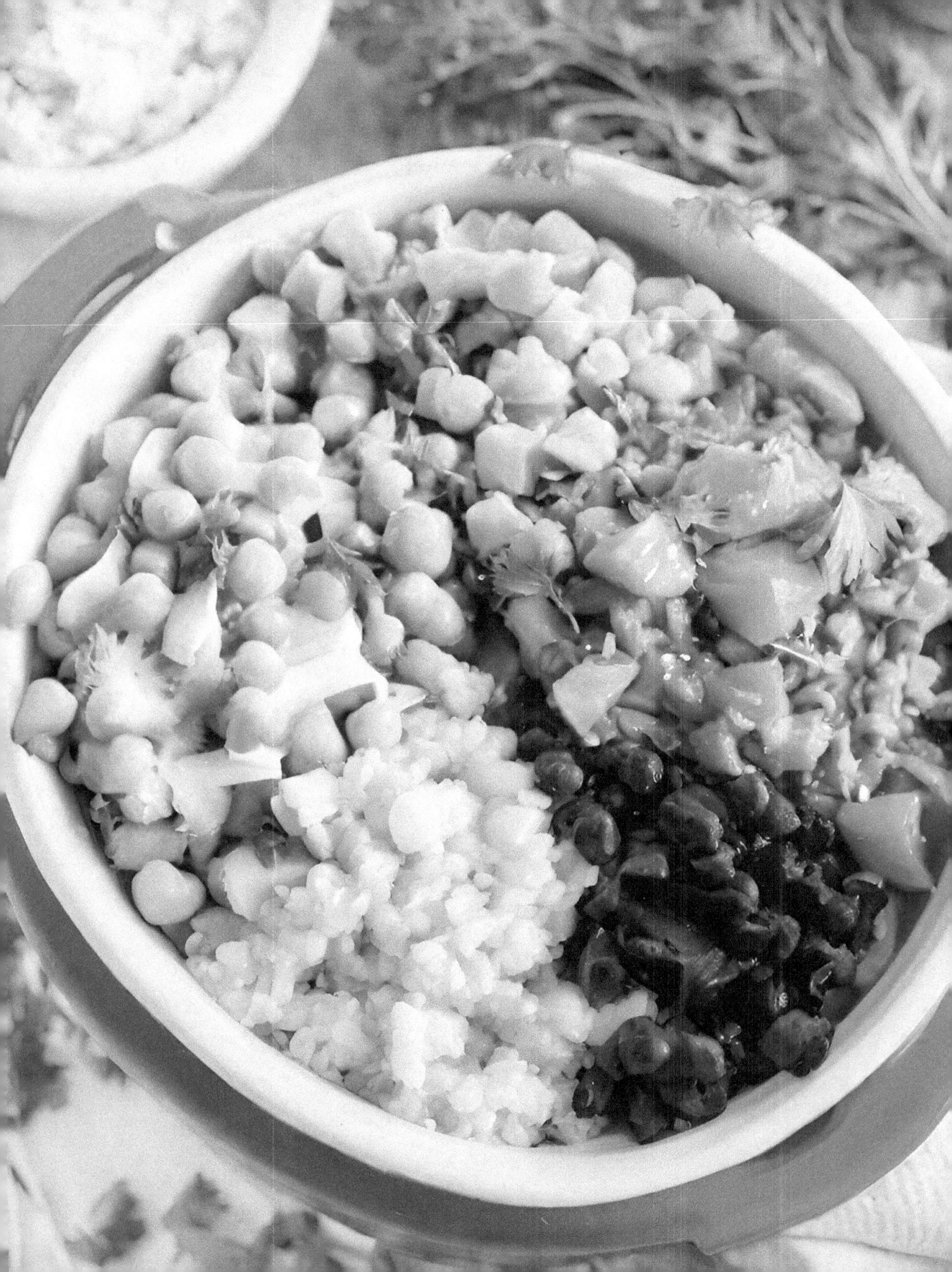

"Introduce the concept of the "Time Savings" series."

"A Culinary Journey Through the Seasons" has been a delightful ride, featuring a diverse collection of crockpot recipes in four volumes. Our readers have explored Asian flavors, relished in meaty delights, embraced vegan-friendly creations, and mastered budget-friendly dishes. But now, it's time to take it a step further with our fifth installment, the "Time Savings" series.

In the "Time Savings" series, we continue our commitment to providing you with mouthwatering crockpot recipes, but with an emphasis on efficiency and convenience. We understand that in today's fast-paced world, time is a valuable commodity. That's why we're here to show you how to create delectable dishes in your crockpot without the hassle.

Each recipe in this series is designed to help you maximize the minutes in your day. With minimal hands-on effort, you can set up your crockpot, go about your business, and return to a savory, perfectly cooked meal. We want to make your cooking experience as efficient as it is delicious.

So, as we delve into the "Time Savings" series, rest assured that the culinary journey continues, now with an added focus on saving you precious time in the kitchen. Whether you're a seasoned chef or a busy homemaker, these recipes are designed to make your life easier while satisfying your taste buds. Let's embark on this journey of quick and efficient crockpot cooking together!

"Emphasize the focus on quick and efficient crockpot cooking."

In the "Time Savings" series, our primary focus is on making crockpot cooking quick, efficient, and hassle-free. We understand that time is precious, and spending hours in the kitchen isn't always an option. That's why each recipe in this series is thoughtfully crafted to minimize your hands-on time and maximize your satisfaction.

With our recipes, you'll find that the crockpot can be your best ally when it comes to saving time in the kitchen. These dishes are perfect for those days when you have a busy schedule, but you still want to enjoy a homemade meal that's bursting with flavor. We'll show you how to make the most of your crockpot, allowing you to prep your ingredients, set the timer, and go about your day while your meal simmers to perfection.

So, if you're searching for ways to make cooking a breeze without compromising on taste, you've come to the right place. Our "Time Savings" series is all about giving you back valuable time in your day while indulging in dishes that will leave your taste buds delighted. Let's explore the world of efficient crockpot cooking together!

""Encourage readers to explore the time-saving recipes in this volume."

"Whether you're a busy professional, a parent juggling multiple responsibilities, or simply someone who values their time, we invite you to dive into the world of time-saving crockpot cooking. Our "Time Savings" series is tailor-made for those who appreciate the efficiency of a crockpot without sacrificing flavor and quality.

These recipes are your answer to delicious, home-cooked meals that don't demand hours of your day. We want you to savor the taste of a lovingly prepared dish without feeling tied to the stove. Let your crockpot do the work while you focus on what matters most to you.

In this volume, you'll find a wide array of recipes that cater to a variety of tastes and preferences. From hearty stews to succulent meat dishes and delightful desserts, we've got your culinary needs covered. The best part? They won't keep you stuck in the kitchen.

So, embark on this culinary journey with us. We encourage you to explore these time-saving recipes and discover the joy of quick and efficient crockpot cooking. Make your life easier while treating your taste buds to scrumptious delights. It's time to enjoy the luxury of time in your busy schedule without compromising on your love for good food."

Chapter 1: Quick and Easy Breakfasts

- **Overnight Oats with Berries**
- **Crockpot Breakfast Casserole**
- **Apple Cinnamon Porridge**
- **Veggie Omelette**
- **Blueberry French Toast**

1. Overnight Oats with Berries

List of Ingredients:

- 2 cups old-fashioned rolled oats
- 2 cups almond milk (or your preferred milk)
- 1/4 cup honey or maple syrup
- 1 cup mixed berries (strawberries, blueberries, raspberries)
- 1/4 cup chopped nuts (almonds, walnuts)
- 1 teaspoon vanilla extract
- 1/2 teaspoon cinnamon

Nutrition Benefits:

This recipe is packed with fiber from oats and antioxidants from mixed berries. It provides a healthy dose of nutrients and energy to start your day.

Calories Count per Serving: Approximately 300 calories per serving.

Time Required:

5 minutes prep time, 6-8 hours cooking time (overnight)

Step-by-Step Instruction:

1. In the crockpot, combine oats, almond milk, honey (or maple syrup), vanilla extract, and cinnamon.
2. Stir well and add the mixed berries.
3. Cover and cook on the low setting for 6-8 hours or overnight.
4. In the morning, give it a good stir, and serve with chopped nuts as toppings.

2. Crockpot Breakfast Casserole

List of Ingredients:

- **6 eggs**
- **2 cups diced ham or turkey sausage**
- **2 cups frozen diced hash browns**
- **1 1/2 cups shredded cheddar cheese**
- **1/2 cup milk**
- **Salt and pepper to taste**
- **Chopped green onions (optional)**

Nutrition Benefits:

This casserole is a protein-packed breakfast with the addition of ham or sausage. It provides essential nutrients to keep you full and satisfied.

Calories Count per Serving: Approximately 350 calories per serving.

Time Required:

15 minutes prep time, 4 hours cooking time

Step-by-Step Instruction:

1. **In a large mixing bowl, beat the eggs and milk together. Add salt and pepper to taste.**
2. **Grease the crockpot and add a layer of diced hash browns.**
3. **Sprinkle half of the ham or sausage on top of the hash browns.**
4. **Add half of the shredded cheddar cheese.**
5. **Repeat with another layer of hash browns, ham (or sausage), and cheese.**
6. **Pour the egg mixture evenly over the layers.**
7. **Cover and cook on the low setting for about 4 hours.**
8. **Sprinkle chopped green onions on top (if desired) before serving.**

3. Apple Cinnamon Porridge

List of Ingredients:

- 2 cups steel-cut oats
- 4 cups water
- 4 cups unsweetened apple juice
- 2 apples, peeled, cored, and diced
- 1/4 cup brown sugar
- 1 teaspoon cinnamon
- A pinch of salt
- Chopped nuts and raisins for topping

Nutrition Benefits:

This porridge is rich in fiber and provides a good amount of natural sugars from apples. It's a warm and comforting breakfast option.

Calories Count per Serving: Approximately 250 calories per serving.

Time Required:

10 minutes prep time, 4 hours cooking time

Step-by-Step Instruction:

1. In the crockpot, combine steel-cut oats, water, unsweetened apple juice, diced apples, brown sugar, cinnamon, and a pinch of salt.
2. Stir well.
3. Cover and cook on the low setting for about 4 hours.
4. Serve hot with chopped nuts and raisins on top.

4. Veggie Omelette

List of Ingredients:

- **8 eggs**
- **1/2 cup milk**
- **1 cup diced bell peppers (red, green, and yellow)**
- **1/2 cup diced onions**
- **1/2 cup diced tomatoes**
- **1/2 cup diced spinach**
- **1 cup shredded cheese (cheddar or your choice)**
- **Salt and pepper to taste**

Nutrition Benefits:

This veggie-packed omelette provides essential vitamins, minerals, and protein, making it a nutritious choice.

Calories Count per Serving: Approximately 250 calories per serving.

Time Required:

10 minutes prep time, 2 hours cooking time

Step-by-Step Instruction:

1. In a bowl, beat the eggs, milk, and add salt and pepper to taste.
2. Grease the crockpot and add the diced bell peppers, onions, tomatoes, and spinach.
3. Pour the egg mixture over the veggies.
4. Sprinkle shredded cheese on top.
5. Cover and cook on the low setting for about 2 hours.
6. Slice into wedges and serve.

5. Blueberry French Toast

List of Ingredients:

- **1 loaf of bread, sliced**
- **2 cups fresh or frozen blueberries**
- **8 eggs**
- **2 cups milk**
- **1/2 cup maple syrup**
- **1 teaspoon vanilla extract**
- **1 teaspoon cinnamon**
- **A pinch of salt**

Nutrition Benefits:

This delicious French toast provides a fruity twist with blueberries and offers a dose of fiber and antioxidants.

Calories Count per Serving: Approximately 300 calories per serving.

Time Required:

15 minutes prep time, 2 hours cooking time

Step-by-Step Instruction:

1. In a bowl, beat the eggs, milk, maple syrup, vanilla extract, cinnamon, and a pinch of salt.
2. Grease the crockpot and place a layer of sliced bread at the bottom.
3. Add a layer of blueberries.
4. Pour half of the egg mixture over the berries and bread.
5. Repeat with another layer of bread, berries, and the remaining egg mixture.
6. Cover and cook on the low setting for about 2 hours.
7. Serve with extra maple syrup.

Chapter 2: Effortless Soups and Stews

1. Hearty Chicken Noodle Soup

List of Ingredients:

- 4 boneless, skinless chicken breasts
- 8 cups chicken broth
- 4 carrots, sliced
- 4 celery stalks, sliced
- 1 onion, chopped
- 3 cloves garlic, minced
- 2 cups egg noodles
- 1 teaspoon dried thyme
- Salt and pepper to taste

Nutrition Benefits:

This comforting soup is packed with lean protein, vegetables, and warming flavors, making it a nourishing choice.

Calories Count per Serving: Approximately 250 calories per serving.

Time Required:

15 minutes prep time, 4 hours cooking time

Step-by-Step Instruction:

1. Place the chicken breasts, chicken broth, carrots, celery, onion, garlic, and dried thyme in the crockpot.
2. Season with salt and pepper.
3. Cover and cook on the low setting for about 4 hours.
4. Remove the chicken, shred it, and return it to the soup.
5. Add the egg noodles and cook for an additional 15-20 minutes or until noodles are tender.

2. Vegetable Lentil Soup

List of Ingredients:

- 1 cup dried green or brown lentils
- 8 cups vegetable broth
- 2 cups diced carrots
- 2 cups diced celery
- 1 onion, chopped
- 2 cloves garlic, minced
- 1 teaspoon cumin
- 1 teaspoon paprika
- Salt and pepper to taste

Nutrition Benefits:

This hearty soup provides a good source of plant-based protein, fiber, and essential nutrients.

Calories Count per Serving: Approximately 220 calories per serving.

Time Required:

15 minutes prep time, 6 hours cooking time

Step-by-Step Instruction:

1. Combine lentils, vegetable broth, carrots, celery, onion, garlic, cumin, paprika, salt, and pepper in the crockpot.
2. Stir well.
3. Cover and cook on the low setting for about 6 hours.

3. Beef and Barley Stew

List of Ingredients:

- 1 pound beef stew meat, cubed
- 1 cup barley
- 8 cups beef broth
- 2 cups sliced mushrooms
- 1 cup diced onions
- 2 cloves garlic, minced
- 2 cups sliced carrots
- 2 cups sliced celery
- 1 teaspoon dried thyme
- Salt and pepper to taste

Nutrition Benefits:

This hearty stew offers protein from beef and the health benefits of barley, making it a nutritious choice.

Calories Count per Serving: Approximately 350 calories per serving.

Time Required:

15 minutes prep time, 6 hours cooking time

Step-by-Step Instruction:

1. Combine beef stew meat, barley, beef broth, mushrooms, onions, garlic, carrots, celery, dried thyme, salt, and pepper in the crockpot.
2. Stir well.
3. Cover and cook on the low setting for about 6 hours.

4. Sweet Potato and Black Bean Chili

List of Ingredients:

- 2 sweet potatoes, peeled and diced
- 2 cans black beans, drained and rinsed
- 2 cans diced tomatoes
- 1 onion, chopped
- 2 cloves garlic, minced
- 2 cups vegetable broth
- 2 tablespoons chili powder
- 1 teaspoon cumin
- Salt and pepper to taste

Nutrition Benefits:

This chili is loaded with fiber, antioxidants, and vitamins from sweet potatoes and black beans.

Calories Count per Serving: Approximately 270 calories per serving.

Time Required:

15 minutes prep time, 4 hours cooking time

Step-by-Step Instruction:

1. Place sweet potatoes, black beans, diced tomatoes, onion, garlic, vegetable broth, chili powder, cumin, salt, and pepper in the crockpot.
2. Stir well.
3. Cover and cook on the low setting for about 4 hours.

5. Creamy Tomato Basil Soup

List of Ingredients:

- **2 cans diced tomatoes**
- **2 cups vegetable broth**
- **1 cup diced onions**
- **2 cloves garlic, minced**
- **1/2 cup fresh basil leaves, chopped**
- **1 cup heavy cream**
- **Salt and pepper to taste**
-

Nutrition Benefits:
This creamy soup offers the delightful flavor of fresh basil and the richness of tomatoes and cream.

Calories Count per Serving: Approximately 280 calories per serving.

Time Required:

15 minutes prep time, 4 hours cooking time

Step-by-Step Instruction:

1. Combine diced tomatoes, vegetable broth, onions, garlic, fresh basil, heavy cream, salt, and pepper in the crockpot.
2. Stir well.
3. Cover and cook on the low setting for about 4 hours.
4. These recipes provide you with quick and delicious soups and stews, saving you time in the kitchen. Enjoy!

Chapter 3: Speedy Chicken Dishes

- **Lemon Garlic Chicken**
- **Honey Sriracha Chicken**
- **BBQ Pulled Chicken**
- **Chicken and Rice Casserole**
- **Creamy Chicken Alfredo**

1. Lemon Garlic Chicken

List of Ingredients:

- 4 boneless, skinless chicken breasts
- 1 lemon, juiced and zested
- 4 cloves garlic, minced
- 1 cup chicken broth
- 1 teaspoon dried thyme
- Salt and pepper to taste
-

Nutrition Benefits:

This dish is low in calories and offers the zesty flavor of lemon along with the health benefits of garlic.

Calories Count per Serving: Approximately 220 calories per serving.

Time Required:

15 minutes prep time, 4 hours cooking time

Step-by-Step Instruction:
1. Place chicken breasts, lemon juice, lemon zest, garlic, chicken broth, dried thyme, salt, and pepper in the crockpot.
2. Cover and cook on the low setting for about 4 hours.

2. Honey Sriracha Chicken

List of Ingredients:

- **4 boneless, skinless chicken thighs**
- **1/4 cup honey**
- **2 tablespoons sriracha sauce**
- **2 tablespoons soy sauce**
- **1 tablespoon rice vinegar**
- **1 clove garlic, minced**
- **Sesame seeds for garnish**

Nutrition Benefits:

This dish combines the sweetness of honey with a touch of heat from sriracha, providing a unique flavor profile.

Calories Count per Serving: Approximately 230 calories per serving.

Time Required:

10 minutes prep time, 3 hours cooking time

Step-by-Step Instruction:

- **In a bowl, whisk together honey, sriracha sauce, soy sauce, rice vinegar, and minced garlic.**
- **Place chicken thighs in the crockpot.**
- **Pour the honey sriracha sauce over the chicken.**
- **Cover and cook on the low setting for about 3 hours.**
- **Garnish with sesame seeds before serving.**

3. BBQ Pulled Chicken

List of Ingredients:

- 4 boneless, skinless chicken breasts
- 1 cup barbecue sauce
- 1/4 cup apple cider vinegar
- 1/4 cup brown sugar
- 1 tablespoon Dijon mustard
- 1/2 teaspoon smoked paprika
- Salt and pepper to taste

Nutrition Benefits:

This dish offers a smoky and tangy barbecue flavor with lean protein from chicken.

Calories Count per Serving: Approximately 260 calories per serving.

Time Required: 10 minutes prep time, 4 hours cooking time

Step-by-Step Instruction:

- Place chicken breasts in the crockpot.
- In a bowl, combine barbecue sauce, apple cider vinegar, brown sugar, Dijon mustard, smoked paprika, salt, and pepper.
- Pour the barbecue sauce mixture over the chicken.
- Cover and cook on the low setting for about 4 hours.
- Shred the chicken before serving.

4. Chicken and Rice Casserole

List of Ingredients:

- 4 boneless, skinless chicken breasts
- 2 cups long-grain rice
- 1 cup chicken broth
- 1 cup sliced mushrooms
- 1 cup diced onions
- 2 cloves garlic, minced
- 1 teaspoon dried thyme
- Salt and pepper to taste

Nutrition Benefits:

This casserole combines chicken, rice, and vegetables for a balanced meal.

Calories Count per Serving: Approximately 290 calories per serving.

Time Required:

15 minutes prep time, 4 hours cooking time

Step-by-Step Instruction:

1. Place chicken breasts, long-grain rice, chicken broth, mushrooms, onions, garlic, dried thyme, salt, and pepper in the crockpot.
2. Stir well.
3. Cover and cook on the low setting for about 4 hours.

5. Creamy Chicken Alfredo

List of Ingredients:

- **4 boneless, skinless chicken thighs**
- **2 cups heavy cream**
- **1 cup grated Parmesan cheese**
- **1/4 cup butter**
- **1/4 cup cream cheese**
- **2 cloves garlic, minced**
- **Salt and pepper to taste**
- **8 oz fettuccine pasta**

Nutrition Benefits:

This dish is rich and indulgent, offering the creamy goodness of Alfredo sauce.

Calories Count per Serving: Approximately 400 calories per serving.

Time Required:

15 minutes prep time, 3 hours cooking time

Step-by-Step Instruction:

1. In a saucepan, combine heavy cream, grated Parmesan cheese, butter, cream cheese, minced garlic, salt, and pepper. Heat and stir until the sauce is smooth.
2. Place chicken thighs in the crockpot.
3. Pour the Alfredo sauce over the chicken.
4. Cover and cook on the low setting for about 3 hours.
5. Cook fettuccine pasta separately according to package instructions and serve the chicken Alfredo over pasta.

Enjoy these quick and delicious chicken dishes prepared in your crockpot!

Chapter 4: Time-Efficient Beef and Pork Creations

- **Beef and Broccoli Stir Fry**
- **Classic Pot Roast**
- **BBQ Pork Ribs**
- **Beef and Vegetable Soup**
- **Teriyaki Beef Tips**

1. Beef and Broccoli Stir Fry

List of Ingredients:

- **1.5 lbs beef sirloin, thinly sliced**
- **2 cups broccoli florets**
- **1/2 cup low-sodium soy sauce**
- **1/4 cup brown sugar**
- **2 cloves garlic, minced**
- **1 teaspoon ginger, grated**
- **1 tablespoon cornstarch**
- **Sesame seeds for garnish**
- **Cooked rice or noodles (for serving)**

Nutrition Benefits:

This dish combines lean beef and broccoli in a savory stir-fry sauce.

Calories Count per Serving: Approximately 350 calories per serving (excluding rice or noodles).

Time Required:

15 minutes prep time, 4 hours cooking time

Step-by-Step Instruction:

1. Place beef slices and broccoli florets in the crockpot.
2. In a bowl, whisk together soy sauce, brown sugar, minced garlic, grated ginger, and cornstarch.
3. Pour the sauce over the beef and broccoli.
4. Cover and cook on the low setting for about 4 hours.
5. Serve over cooked rice or noodles and garnish with sesame seeds.

2. Classic Pot Roast

List of Ingredients:

- **2.5 lbs chuck roast**
- **4 carrots, peeled and sliced**
- **4 potatoes, peeled and cubed**
- **1 onion, chopped**
- **2 cups beef broth**
- **1 packet of onion soup mix**
- **Salt and pepper to taste**

Nutrition Benefits:

This hearty pot roast combines tender beef with classic vegetables.

Calories Count per Serving: Approximately 400 calories per serving.

Time Required:

15 minutes prep time, 7-8 hours cooking time

Step-by-Step Instruction:

1. Place chuck roast, carrots, potatoes, and chopped onion in the crockpot.

2. In a bowl, mix together beef broth and onion soup mix.

3. Pour the mixture over the ingredients in the crockpot.

4. Season with salt and pepper.

5. Cover and cook on the low setting for 7-8 hours.

3. BBQ Pork Ribs

List of Ingredients:

- **2 lbs pork ribs**
- **1 cup barbecue sauce**
- **1/4 cup apple cider vinegar**
- **1/4 cup brown sugar**
- **1/2 teaspoon paprika**
- **1/2 teaspoon chili powder**
- **Salt and pepper to taste**

Nutrition Benefits:

These succulent BBQ pork ribs are perfect for a flavorful feast.

Calories Count per Serving: Approximately 350 calories per serving.

Time Required:

15 minutes prep time, 4 hours cooking time

Step-by-Step Instruction:

1. Cut the pork ribs into serving-size pieces and place them in the crockpot.
2. In a bowl, combine barbecue sauce, apple cider vinegar, brown sugar, paprika, chili powder, salt, and pepper.
3. Pour the sauce over the ribs.
4. Cover and cook on the low setting for about 4 hours.

4. Beef and Vegetable Soup

List of Ingredients:

- **1.5 lbs beef stew meat, cubed**
- **4 cups beef broth**
- **1 onion, chopped**
- **2 carrots, sliced**
- **2 potatoes, peeled and cubed**
- **1 cup frozen peas**
- **1 cup frozen corn**
- **2 cloves garlic, minced**
- **1 teaspoon thyme**
- **Salt and pepper to taste**

Nutrition Benefits:

This hearty soup is packed with beef and a variety of vegetables.

Calories Count per Serving: Approximately 250 calories per serving.

Time Required:

15 minutes prep time, 7-8 hours cooking time

Step-by-Step Instruction:

1. Place beef stew meat, chopped onion, sliced carrots, cubed potatoes, frozen peas, frozen corn, minced garlic, thyme, salt, and pepper in the crockpot.
2. Add beef broth to the crockpot.
3. Cover and cook on the low setting for 7-8 hours.

5. Teriyaki Beef Tips

List of Ingredients:

- **1.5 lbs beef tips or sirloin, cubed**
- **1/2 cup soy sauce**
- **1/4 cup brown sugar**
- **1/4 cup pineapple juice**
- **2 cloves garlic, minced**
- **1 teaspoon ginger, grated**
- **1 tablespoon cornstarch**
- **Sesame seeds and sliced green onions for garnish**
- **Cooked rice (for serving)**

Nutrition Benefits:

These teriyaki beef tips offer a delightful blend of sweet and savory flavors.

Calories Count per Serving: Approximately 320 calories per serving (excluding rice).

Time Required:

15 minutes prep time, 4 hours cooking time

Step-by-Step Instruction:

1. Place beef tips in the crockpot.
2. In a bowl, whisk together soy sauce, brown sugar, pineapple juice, minced garlic, grated ginger, and cornstarch.
3. Pour the teriyaki sauce over the beef tips.
4. Cover and cook on the low setting for about 4 hours.
5. Serve over cooked rice and garnish with sesame seeds and sliced green onions.

These time-efficient beef and pork creations are perfect for delicious and hassle-free meals. Enjoy!

Chapter 5: Rapid Seafood Meals

- **Lemon Butter Garlic Shrimp**

- **Crockpot Salmon with Herbs**

- **Spicy Seafood Gumbo**

- **Clam Chowder**

- **Tilapia with Mediterranean Veggies**

1. Lemon Butter Garlic Shrimp

List of Ingredients:

- 1 lb large shrimp, peeled and deveined
- 4 cloves garlic, minced
- 1/4 cup unsalted butter, melted
- Zest and juice of 1 lemon
- 1/4 teaspoon red pepper flakes (optional)
- Salt and pepper to taste
- Fresh parsley, chopped (for garnish)
- Cooked rice or pasta (for serving)

Nutrition Benefits:

This shrimp dish offers a burst of citrusy flavors with the goodness of garlic.

Calories Count per Serving: Approximately 200 calories per serving (excluding rice or pasta).

Time Required:

10 minutes prep time, 1.5 hours cooking time

Step-by-Step Instruction:

1. Place peeled and deveined shrimp in the crockpot.
2. In a bowl, combine minced garlic, melted butter, lemon zest, lemon juice, red pepper flakes (if using), salt, and pepper.
3. Pour the mixture over the shrimp.
4. Cover and cook on the low setting for about 1.5 hours.
5. Serve over cooked rice or pasta, garnished with fresh parsley.

2. Crockpot Salmon with Herbs

List of Ingredients:

- **4 salmon fillets**
- **1 lemon, sliced**
- **2 cloves garlic, minced**
- **1 teaspoon dried thyme**
- **1 teaspoon dried rosemary**
- **Salt and pepper to taste**
- **Fresh dill (for garnish)**
- **Cooked quinoa or rice (for serving)**

Nutrition Benefits:

This salmon recipe features a flavorful blend of herbs and citrus.

Calories Count per Serving: Approximately 300 calories per serving (excluding quinoa or rice).

Time Required:

10 minutes prep time, 2 hours cooking time

Step-by-Step Instruction:

1. Place salmon fillets in the crockpot.
2. Lay lemon slices on top of the salmon.
3. In a small bowl, combine minced garlic, dried thyme, dried rosemary, salt, and pepper.
4. Sprinkle the herb mixture evenly over the salmon.
5. Cover and cook on the low setting for about 2 hours.
6. Serve over cooked quinoa or rice, garnished with fresh dill.

3. Spicy Seafood Gumbo

List of Ingredients:

- 1 lb shrimp, peeled and deveined
- 1 lb white fish fillets, cubed
- 1/2 lb andouille sausage, sliced
- 1 onion, chopped
- 1 green bell pepper, chopped
- 2 stalks celery, chopped
- 3 cloves garlic, minced
- 1 can (14 oz) diced tomatoes
- 4 cups seafood or chicken broth
- 1 teaspoon dried thyme
- 1 teaspoon Cajun seasoning
- Salt and pepper to taste
- Cooked rice (for serving)
- Chopped green onions (for garnish)

Nutrition Benefits:

This spicy seafood gumbo is a hearty and satisfying dish with a hint of Cajun spice.

Calories Count per Serving: Approximately 350 calories per serving (excluding rice).

Time Required:

15 minutes prep time, 3-4 hours cooking time

Step-by-Step Instruction:

1. In the crockpot, combine peeled and deveined shrimp, cubed white fish, sliced andouille sausage, chopped onion, chopped green bell pepper, chopped celery, minced garlic, diced tomatoes, seafood or chicken broth, dried thyme, Cajun seasoning, salt, and pepper.
2. Cover and cook on the low setting for 3-4 hours.
3. Serve over cooked rice, garnished with chopped green onions.

4. Clam Chowder

List of Ingredients:

- **2 cans (10 oz each) minced clams, undrained**
- **2 cups potatoes, peeled and diced**
- **1 onion, chopped**
- **1 cup celery, chopped**
- **2 cups vegetable broth**
- **1 teaspoon dried thyme**
- **1 teaspoon dried parsley**
- **1/2 teaspoon garlic powder**
- **Salt and pepper to taste**
- **1 cup half-and-half**
- **Cooked bacon bits (for garnish, optional)**

Nutrition Benefits:

This creamy clam chowder combines tender clams, vegetables, and herbs in a rich broth.

Calories Count per Serving: Approximately 250 calories per serving.

Time Required:

15 minutes prep time, 3-4 hours cooking time

Step-by-Step Instruction:

1. In the crockpot, combine minced clams (with juice), diced potatoes, chopped onion, chopped celery, vegetable broth, dried thyme, dried parsley, garlic powder, salt, and pepper.
2. Cover and cook on the low setting for 3-4 hours until the potatoes are tender.
3. Stir in half-and-half.
4. Serve hot, garnished with cooked bacon bits if desired.

5. Tilapia with Mediterranean Veggies

List of Ingredients:

- 4 tilapia fillets
- 1 cup cherry tomatoes, halved
- 1 zucchini, sliced
- 1 yellow bell pepper, sliced
- 1/2 red onion, sliced
- 3 cloves garlic, minced
- 1 teaspoon dried oregano
- 1 teaspoon dried basil
- Salt and pepper to taste
- 1 lemon, sliced
- Fresh parsley (for garnish)
- Cooked quinoa or rice (for serving)

Nutrition Benefits:

This tilapia recipe combines Mediterranean flavors with the mild taste of fish.

Calories Count per Serving: Approximately 200 calories per serving (excluding quinoa or rice).

Time Required:

10 minutes prep time, 2 hours cooking time

Step-by-Step Instruction:

1. Place tilapia fillets in the crockpot.
2. In a bowl, combine halved cherry tomatoes, sliced zucchini, sliced yellow bell pepper, sliced red onion, minced garlic, dried oregano, dried basil, salt, and pepper.
3. Pour the veggie mixture over the tilapia.
4. Lay lemon slices on top.
5. Cover and cook on the low setting for about 2 hours.
6. Serve over cooked quinoa or rice, garnished with fresh parsley.

Conclusion:

- Summarize the variety of time-saving crockpot recipes included in this volume.
- Encourage readers to enjoy quick and delicious meals not only during Croctober but throughout the year.

Bonus Section: Create Your Own Recipes!

We Include Blank Recipe Cards Templates and Notes Sections for Your Own Cooking Journals. Be Creative. Explore the Endless Possibilities and Create Your Own. Feel Free to Reproduce the Templates for your Own Use.

"Summary the variety of time-saving crockpot recipes included in this volume:"

In this volume, you've discovered a delightful array of time-saving crockpot recipes designed to make your life in the kitchen easier without compromising on flavor. From quick and easy breakfasts to effortless soups, stews, and a variety of speedy main dishes, these recipes offer the perfect blend of convenience and deliciousness.

You'll find yourself preparing mouthwatering meals without the usual hassle, leaving you with more time to savor and enjoy the culinary creations you've effortlessly prepared. Whether you're a seasoned home chef or just looking for a way to whip up delightful dishes without spending hours in the kitchen, the recipes in this volume will become your go-to time-saving solution.

So, dive in, explore these time-efficient recipes, and experience the joy of savoring a home-cooked meal that's kind to your schedule. Say goodbye to kitchen stress and hello to delightful dining—because great food doesn't have to mean great effort.

Enjoy these recipes year-round, save time, and satisfy your taste buds while doing it.

Happy cooking!

Encourage readers to enjoy quick and delicious meals not only during Croctober but throughout the year:

While these recipes are perfect for Croctober and your fall and winter months, they're designed to bring time-saving joy to your kitchen all year round. Don't limit yourself to just one season; let the convenience of crockpot cooking enhance your culinary adventures throughout the year.

Whether you're a busy student, a working professional, a parent juggling many responsibilities, or anyone who appreciates delicious meals without the fuss, these time-saving recipes will be your trusted companions for all seasons. From hearty breakfasts to savory soups, and speedy main courses to delightful desserts, you'll find the perfect recipe for every occasion and time constraint.

So, let's embrace the wonderful world of quick and delicious cooking, leaving you more time to enjoy your creations and the moments that matter most.

Happy crockpot cooking year-round!

Bonus Section: Create Your Own Recipes!

In the spirit of culinary exploration and creativity, we're excited to offer you a bonus section that's sure to spark your inner chef. Inside, you'll find blank recipe card templates and notes sections, just waiting for your culinary inspiration to take flight.

Cooking is not only about following recipes but also about inventing new ones. With these templates at your fingertips, you can document your own culinary creations, jot down your unique flavor combinations, and craft personalized masterpieces in the kitchen. There are no boundaries here—feel free to experiment, adapt, and make these templates your own.

So, be bold, be inventive, and create dishes that reflect your taste and style. Explore the endless possibilities, and let your inner chef shine. Whether you're a seasoned pro or just starting your culinary journey, these templates are your canvas for flavorful adventures.

Happy cooking, and may your kitchen be a place of endless culinary exploration!

Recipe Card

| NAME OF RECIPE | INGREDIENTS |

SERVE

2 4 6 8

DIFFICULTY

Vegetarian ☐
Dairy Free ☐
Low Carb ☐
Sugar Free ☐
Low Salt ☐

TIME TO PREPARE

REVIEW

INGREDIENTS

INSTRUCTIONS

Recipe Card

NAME OF RECIPE	INGREDIENTS

SERVE

2   4   6   8

DIFFICULTY

Vegetarian ☐
Dairy Free ☐
Low Carb ☐
Sugar Free ☐
Low Salt ☐

TIME TO PREPARE

REVIEW

INSTRUCTIONS

Recipe Card

| NAME OF RECIPE | INGREDIENTS |

SERVE

| 2 | 4 | 6 | 8 |

DIFFICULTY

Vegetarian ☐
Dairy Free ☐
Low Carb ☐
Sugar Free ☐
Low Salt ☐

TIME TO PREPARE

REVIEW

INSTRUCTIONS

Recipe Card

| NAME OF RECIPE | INGREDIENTS |

SERVE

| 2 | 4 | 6 | 8 |

DIFFICULTY

Vegetarian ☐
Dairy Free ☐
Low Carb ☐
Sugar Free ☐
Low Salt ☐

TIME TO PREPARE

REVIEW

INSTRUCTIONS

Recipe Card

NAME OF RECIPE	INGREDIENTS

SERVE

2 · 4 · 6 · 8

DIFFICULTY

INSTRUCTIONS

Vegetarian ☐
Dairy Free ☐
Low Carb ☐
Sugar Free ☐
Low Salt ☐

TIME TO PREPARE

REVIEW

Recipe Card

NAME OF RECIPE	INGREDIENTS

....

SERVE

2 4 6 8

....

DIFFICULTY

....

Vegetarian	☐
Dairy Free	☐
Low Carb	☐
Sugar Free	☐
Low Salt	☐

TIME TO PREPARE

....

REVIEW

INSTRUCTIONS

Recipe Card

NAME OF RECIPE	INGREDIENTS

SERVE

2 4 6 8

DIFFICULTY

- Vegetarian ☐
- Dairy Free ☐
- Low Carb ☐
- Sugar Free ☐
- Low Salt ☐

TIME TO PREPARE

REVIEW

INSTRUCTIONS

Recipe Card

| NAME OF RECIPE | INGREDIENTS |

....

SERVE

| 2 | 4 | 6 | 8 |

....

DIFFICULTY

....

Vegetarian ☐
Dairy Free ☐
Low Carb ☐
Sugar Free ☐
Low Salt ☐

INSTRUCTIONS

TIME TO PREPARE

....

REVIEW

Recipe Card

| NAME OF RECIPE | INGREDIENTS |

SERVE

2 4 6 8

DIFFICULTY

Vegetarian ☐
Dairy Free ☐
Low Carb ☐
Sugar Free ☐
Low Salt ☐

INSTRUCTIONS

TIME TO PREPARE

REVIEW

Recipe Card

NAME OF RECIPE

INGREDIENTS

SERVE

2   4   6   8

DIFFICULTY

INSTRUCTIONS

Vegetarian ☐
Dairy Free ☐
Low Carb ☐
Sugar Free ☐
Low Salt ☐

TIME TO PREPARE

REVIEW

Recipe Card

NAME OF RECIPE	INGREDIENTS

SERVE

2 4 6 8

DIFFICULTY

Vegetarian ☐
Dairy Free ☐
Low Carb ☐
Sugar Free ☐
Low Salt ☐

INSTRUCTIONS

TIME TO PREPARE

REVIEW

Recipe Card

NAME OF RECIPE	INGREDIENTS

SERVE

2　4　6　8

DIFFICULTY

INSTRUCTIONS

Vegetarian ☐
Dairy Free ☐
Low Carb ☐
Sugar Free ☐
Low Salt ☐

TIME TO PREPARE

REVIEW

Recipe Card

NAME OF RECIPE

SERVE

2 4 6 8

DIFFICULTY

Vegetarian ☐
Dairy Free ☐
Low Carb ☐
Sugar Free ☐
Low Salt ☐

TIME TO PREPARE

REVIEW

INGREDIENTS

INSTRUCTIONS

Recipe Card

| NAME OF RECIPE | INGREDIENTS |

SERVE

2   4   6   8

DIFFICULTY

Vegetarian ☐
Dairy Free ☐
Low Carb ☐
Sugar Free ☐
Low Salt ☐

TIME TO PREPARE

REVIEW

INSTRUCTIONS

Recipe Card

| NAME OF RECIPE | INGREDIENTS |

SERVE

2 4 6 8

DIFFICULTY

Vegetarian ☐
Dairy Free ☐
Low Carb ☐
Sugar Free ☐
Low Salt ☐

TIME TO PREPARE

REVIEW

INSTRUCTIONS

Recipe Card

NAME OF RECIPE	INGREDIENTS

SERVE

2   4   6   8

DIFFICULTY

INSTRUCTIONS

Vegetarian ☐
Dairy Free ☐
Low Carb ☐
Sugar Free ☐
Low Salt ☐

TIME TO PREPARE

REVIEW

Recipe Card

NAME OF RECIPE

SERVE

| 2 | 4 | 6 | 8 |

DIFFICULTY

- Vegetarian ☐
- Dairy Free ☐
- Low Carb ☐
- Sugar Free ☐
- Low Salt ☐

TIME TO PREPARE

REVIEW

INGREDIENTS

INSTRUCTIONS

Recipe Card

NAME OF RECIPE

SERVE

| 2 | 4 | 6 | 8 |

DIFFICULTY

Vegetarian ☐
Dairy Free ☐
Low Carb ☐
Sugar Free ☐
Low Salt ☐

TIME TO PREPARE

REVIEW

INGREDIENTS

INSTRUCTIONS

NOTES

Recipe Card

2 4 6 8

Vegetarian ☐
Dairy Free ☐
Low Carb ☐
Sugar Free ☐
Low Salt ☐

NOTES

DATE

Recipe Card

| NAME OF RECIPE | INGREDIENTS |

....

SERVE

| 2 | 4 | 6 | 8 |

....

DIFFICULTY

....

INSTRUCTIONS

Vegetarian ☐
Dairy Free ☐
Low Carb ☐
Sugar Free ☐
Low Salt ☐

TIME TO PREPARE

....

REVIEW

NOTES

DATE

Recipe Card

| NAME OF RECIPE | INGREDIENTS |

SERVE

| 2 | 4 | 6 | 8 |

| DIFFICULTY | INSTRUCTIONS |

Vegetarian ☐
Dairy Free ☐
Low Carb ☐
Sugar Free ☐
Low Salt ☐

TIME TO PREPARE

REVIEW

NOTES

Recipe Card

NOTES

DATE

NOTES

NOTES

DATE

NOTES

DATE

NOTES

NOTES

DATE

NOTES

NOTES

NOTES

DATE

NOTES

DATE

NOTES

NOTES

DATE

NOTES

NOTES

DATE

NOTES

NOTES

NOTES

DATE